A SUGAR-FREE

DIET FOR HEALTHY LIVING

Tailoring a Sugar-Free Lifestyle: Age and Gender Considerations For Optimal Health.

Gracie D. Wolff

TABLE OF CONTENTS:

CHAPTER 1:

INTRODUCTION

Welcome, dear reader, to the insightful journey we are about to embark upon together within the pages of "Tailoring a Sugar-Free Lifestyle: Age and Gender Considerations for Optimal Health." It's not just a guide; it's a roadmap forged from personal experiences, a roadmap that speaks the language of simplicity, devoid of fancy words and complex jargon, designed to be your partner in the quest for better health.

In the era of countless health fads and dietary trends, I found myself standing at a crossroads, grappling with health issues that seemed to defy conventional solutions. It was during this pivotal moment that the curtain lifted on the profound impact sugar could have on our overall well-being. This book is a testament to the transformative power of understanding, adapting, and tailoring a lifestyle to one's unique needs.

Let me take you back to the genesis of this journey, a time when the whispers of change were barely audible amidst the cacophony of daily life. It was a moment that began with introspection, a reflection upon the choices I made, and the consequences they wrought on my health. At the core of this realization was the pervasive influence of sugar, a seemingly innocuous ingredient that, unbeknownst to many, held the key to unlocking a path towards profound well-being.

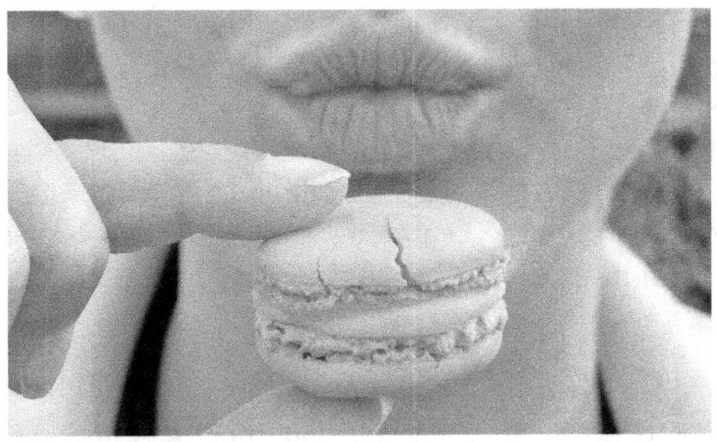

Picture this: a person navigating the labyrinth of health-related challenges, facing issues that seemed elusive to traditional approaches. Through research, trials, and errors, the veil was lifted, revealing the profound impact of sugar on the body and mind. It was not a sudden epiphany but a gradual unraveling of the intricate web woven by the sugar-laden modern diet.

In sharing my personal story, it's not about recounting struggles for the sake of empathy but rather to bridge the gap between my experiences and yours. I am no different from you, and that's the beauty of our shared journey. We are all seekers, explorers on the path to optimal health, and this book is a compass to guide us through the uncharted territories of sugar-free living.

As we delve into the heart of these pages, my aim is not to inundate you with complex theories or esoteric nutritional knowledge. Instead, I offer practical insights, real-world tips, and relatable anecdotes to demystify the process of adopting a sugar-free lifestyle. It's about making informed choices without succumbing to the overwhelming confusion often associated with health-related decisions.

Consider this book a conversation, an intimate dialogue between us where I share not just the 'what' and 'why' but also the 'how.' How can you tailor a sugar-free lifestyle to different ages? How does gender influence this journey? These are the questions we will explore together, and by the end of this journey, you'll not only have answers but a personalized roadmap for your unique path to optimal health.

In the chapters that follow, we'll dissect the intricate relationship between sugar and our bodies, unraveling the often overlooked impacts on different age groups – from the playful energy of childhood to the wisdom of senior years. We'll navigate through the nuances of gender-specific considerations, understanding that health is not a one-size-fits-all equation but a harmonious symphony of individual needs.

But let's not get ahead of ourselves. Before we delve into the nitty-gritty details, let me be clear – this isn't about deprivation or strict regimens. It's a celebration of choices, a journey of empowerment where you are the protagonist, the architect of your health narrative. I'm merely a guide, offering insights garnered from my own expedition, pointing out the landmarks and potential pitfalls to make your journey smoother.

As we explore the practical tips for implementing a sugar-free diet, discover healthier alternatives, and navigate the social landscapes filled with sugary temptations, remember that this journey is not about perfection but progress. It's about embracing the small victories and understanding that every step taken towards a sugar-free lifestyle is a step towards a healthier, more vibrant you.

Recipes and meal plans will be our companions in the kitchen, transforming the notion of 'diet' into a delightful culinary adventure. We'll discuss the crucial role of exercise in the realm of sugar-free living, understanding that movement is not just a physical activity but a holistic approach to well-being.

Monitoring progress and adjusting the plan are integral aspects of this journey. We'll delve into the importance of self-reflection, understanding that our bodies are dynamic entities, ever-changing and responding to the choices we make. Overcoming common obstacles will be a shared exploration, acknowledging that challenges are not roadblocks but opportunities for growth.

And finally, a powerful call to action awaits you at the conclusion of this book. It's not just a conclusion but an invitation – an invitation to take the reins of your health, to implement the knowledge gained, and to shape your future with conscious choices. This book is not the end but a beginning, a catalyst for change, and I implore you to step into the next chapter of your life with newfound determination.

Your journey to a sugar-free lifestyle starts now. As you turn the pages, envision the possibilities, embrace the knowledge, and let this book be your ally in the pursuit of a healthier, more fulfilling life. Together, let's unlock the wonders that lie within – your body's thanksgiving awaits.

CHAPTER 2:

UNDERSTANDING THE IMPACT OF SUGAR ON HEALTH

In the intricate tapestry of our daily lives, sugar often finds its place as a sweet indulgence, adding flavor to our foods and beverages. Little did I realize the profound impact it was silently exerting on my health until I embarked on a journey of understanding. This chapter is not just a collection of facts; it's a revelation born out of personal experience.

Picture this: the typical day, starting with a seemingly innocent bowl of cereal and ending with a sweet treat after dinner. My reliance on sugary comforts was habitual, much like many others navigating the modern food landscape. It wasn't until I began connecting the dots between my energy levels, mood swings, and overall well-being that the silent culprit emerged – sugar.

1. The Sweet Saboteur: Unraveling Sugar's Effects

Sugar, in its various forms, infiltrates our diets with stealth, contributing to a myriad of health issues. One of the most significant impacts is on our energy levels. The initial surge of energy after consuming sugary snacks is nothing more than a fleeting illusion. The subsequent crash leaves us fatigued and craving more, perpetuating a cycle of dependence.

Beyond the energy rollercoaster, sugar has a notorious association with weight gain. The excess calories from added sugars can lead to an imbalance in our energy equation, fostering the accumulation of unwanted pounds. My journey into understanding this wasn't just about shedding physical weight but breaking free from the emotional weight of sugar dependency.

2. Sweet Deception: The Hidden Sugars

Understanding the impact of sugar requires more than just avoiding obvious sources like candy and sodas. It's about unmasking the hidden sugars that lurk in seemingly healthy options. Condiments, salad dressings, and even seemingly wholesome yogurt can harbor substantial amounts of added sugars.

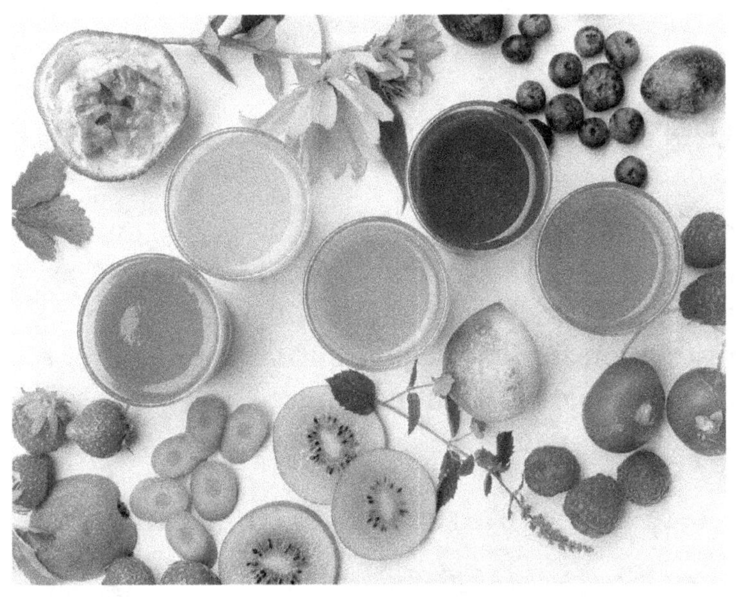

Reading labels became a game-changer in my quest for a healthier lifestyle.

The insidious effects extend beyond the physical realm, infiltrating our mental well-being. Sugar has been linked to mood swings, anxiety, and even cognitive decline. Reflecting on my own experiences, the foggy mental state and erratic emotions began to make sense as I unraveled the connection between my sugar intake and mental health.

CHAPTER 3:

BENEFITS OF A SUGAR-FREE DIET

As the layers of sugar's impact were peeled away, the prospect of a sugar-free lifestyle emerged as a beacon of well-being. This chapter is not a prescription for deprivation but a celebration of the myriad benefits awaiting those who choose to navigate this path.

1. The Sweet Liberation: Breaking Free from Sugar's Grip

One of the most liberating aspects of adopting a sugar-free diet is the newfound sense of control. No longer dictated by the whims of sugar-induced cravings, I discovered a more stable and consistent energy level. The peaks and valleys of my daily vitality became smoother, fostering a sustained sense of well-being.

Weight management took on a new dimension as I embraced the benefits of a sugar-free diet. Shedding the excess pounds wasn't just about appearance; it was about lightening the load on my body, allowing it to function optimally. The scale became a reflection of a holistic approach to health, rather than a mere numerical metric.

2. Clarity of Mind: Unveiling Mental Well-being

Perhaps one of the most profound benefits was the clarity that permeated my mind. The fog lifted, and mental acuity became a constant companion. Research supports the notion that reducing sugar intake can positively impact cognitive function, and my experiences echoed this sentiment.

3. A Sweet Reversal: Combatting Health Issues

As I ventured further into a sugar-free lifestyle, I witnessed a reversal of some health issues that had become unwelcome companions on my journey. From improved dental health to a more robust immune system, the benefits extended beyond the surface. Inflammation levels decreased, and the risk factors for chronic diseases began to diminish.

4. A Taste of True Flavor: Rediscovering Food

One of the unexpected joys of embracing a sugar-free diet was the reawakening of my taste buds. Natural flavors became more vibrant, and a subtle sweetness in fruits and vegetables took center stage. It was a culinary adventure, proving that a sugar-free life is not about deprivation but a journey into a world of authentic, wholesome flavors.

In the pages that follow, these chapters lay the foundation for a profound exploration into tailoring a sugar-free lifestyle. Understanding the impact of sugar is the first step, and the benefits of a sugar-free diet are the driving force propelling us toward optimal health. As we continue this journey, remember that each revelation is a stepping stone, and the path to well-being is paved with informed choices.

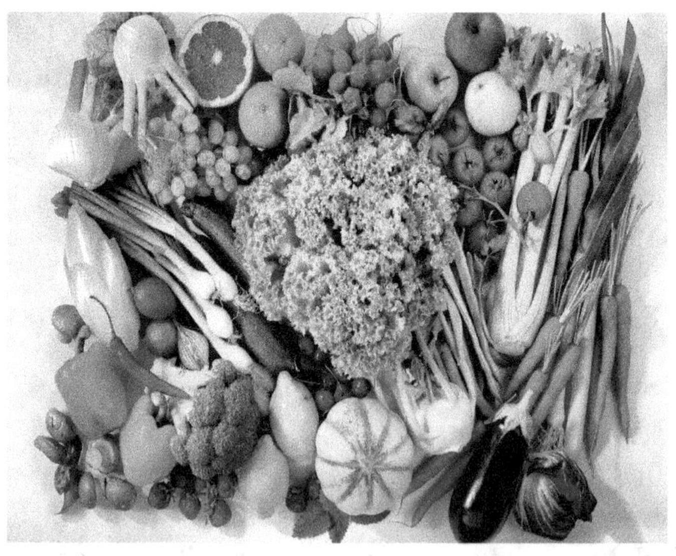

CHAPTER 4:

TAILORING A SUGAR-FREE LIFESTYLE

The journey towards a sugar-free lifestyle is a deeply personal odyssey, marked by unique challenges and triumphs. In this chapter, we'll explore the intricate process of tailoring this lifestyle to suit various age groups and delve into the nuanced considerations based on gender. By understanding the diverse needs of individuals, we can craft a more accessible and sustainable approach to sugar-free living.

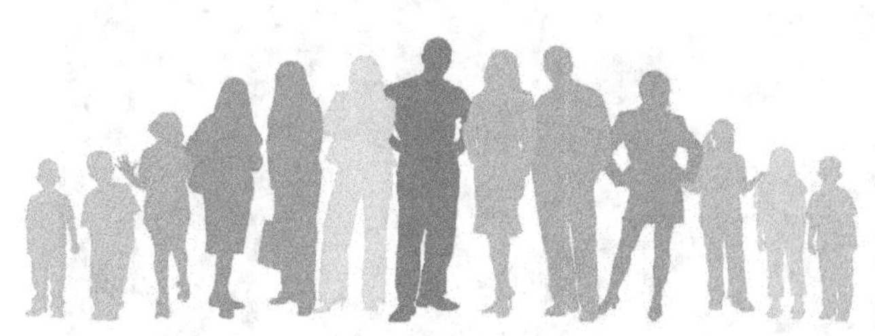

CHAPTER 4.1:

CUSTOMIZING FOR DIFFERENT AGE GROUPS

Our nutritional requirements evolve across the lifespan, from the playful days of childhood to the wisdom-filled senior years. This section delves into the distinctive considerations for each age group.

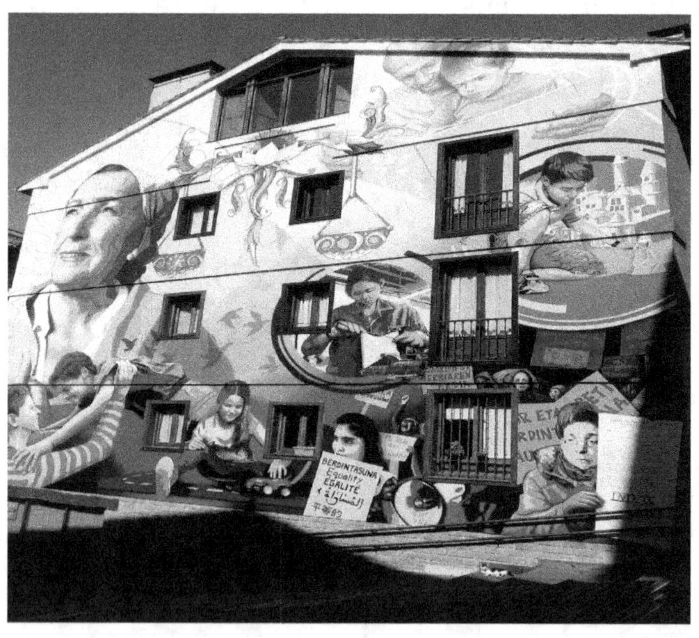

CHAPTER 4.1.1:

CHILDREN AND ADOLESCENTS

Children and adolescents represent a stage of rapid growth and development, making their nutritional needs particularly crucial. Navigating the world of sugar with young ones requires a delicate balance between providing essential nutrients for growth and safeguarding against the potential pitfalls of excessive sugar consumption.

As a parent, my journey into a sugar-free lifestyle involved a keen awareness of the pervasive presence of sugar in children's diets. From cereals marketed as healthy to seemingly innocent fruit-flavored snacks, the battleground against hidden sugars required vigilance. Customizing a sugar-free lifestyle for this age group isn't about deprivation but education.

By introducing the concept of 'smart sweets' and engaging children in the kitchen, we can transform the narrative from restriction to empowerment. Crafting sugar-free treats together becomes an educational journey, fostering a lifelong understanding of nutrition and its impact on overall well-being.

CHAPTER 4.1.2:

ADULTS

Navigating a sugar-free lifestyle in adulthood often involves breaking deeply ingrained habits and reevaluating the role of sugar in daily routines. My own transformation in this phase required a conscious effort to untangle the emotional ties to sugary comfort foods and redefine what constituted a satisfying meal.

For adults, customization revolves around finding a sustainable balance. Experimenting with alternative sweeteners, exploring the vast array of naturally sweet options, and cultivating mindfulness around food choices are integral components. This stage demands a nuanced understanding of social dynamics, where navigating restaurants and social gatherings requires strategic planning without sacrificing enjoyment.

Balancing the practicalities of life with the commitment to a sugar-free lifestyle becomes an art. From meal prepping to smart grocery shopping, adults learn to integrate these practices seamlessly into their daily lives, fostering a sustainable and enjoyable journey towards optimal health.

CHAPTER 4.1.3:

SENIORS

Seniors, in their golden years, encounter unique health considerations that require a tailored approach to a sugar-free lifestyle. Factors such as metabolic changes, potential dietary restrictions, and the desire for optimal well-being underscore the need for customization.

As someone who has delved into this demographic, I've come to appreciate that customization for seniors isn't about imposition but adaptation. Nurturing health through nutrient-dense, sugar-free options becomes a way to support their overall well-being. The focus shifts from restrictive diets to choices that enhance vitality and quality of life.

In this stage, customization is about celebrating the wisdom of the years while navigating the complexities of health. Introducing enjoyable, health-conscious alternatives becomes a way to honor the body's evolving needs and maintain a robust, sugar-free lifestyle.

CHAPTER 4.2:

GENDER-SPECIFIC CONSIDERATIONS

Beyond age, gender-specific considerations add an extra layer of nuance to the sugar-free journey. Recognizing the distinct nutritional needs and challenges faced by men and women enables a more tailored and effective approach.

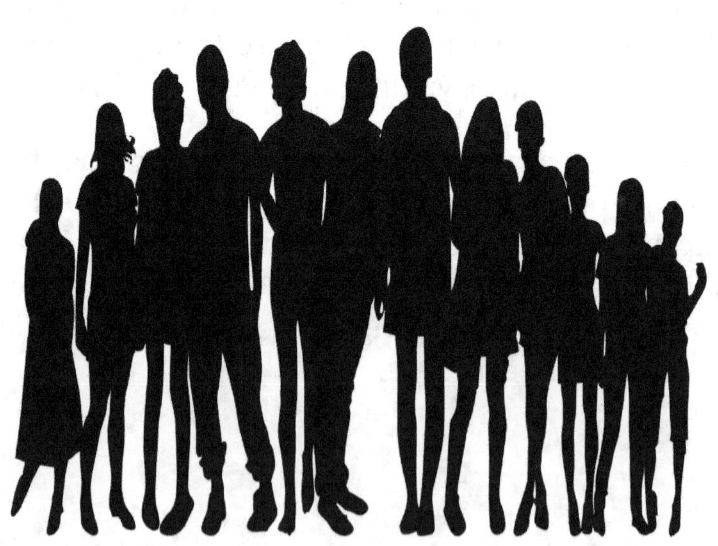

CHAPTER 4.2.1:

MEN

Men, often associated with higher energy expenditure and muscle mass, require a personalized approach to a sugar-free lifestyle. Drawing from my experiences, I've come to understand the significance of incorporating protein-rich, sugar-free options to support physical activity and overall health.

For men, customization involves embracing a diverse array of foods that contribute to a sugar-free lifestyle while meeting their unique nutritional needs. From exploring savory snacks to incorporating robust protein sources, the journey is not just about eliminating sugar but enhancing overall health.

Balancing the dynamic lifestyle of men with the commitment to a sugar-free existence becomes an exploration of possibilities. Recognizing that individual tastes and preferences play a crucial role, men learn to tailor their approach, making the journey not just effective but enjoyable.

CHAPTER 4.2.2:

WOMEN

Women's bodies undergo unique changes, from hormonal fluctuations to distinct nutritional requirements throughout various life stages. As someone who has navigated these intricacies, I've come to appreciate the importance of recognizing and adapting to these dynamics when pursuing a sugar-free lifestyle.

For women, customization often involves addressing specific cravings during different phases of the menstrual cycle and ensuring an adequate intake of essential nutrients. The ebb and flow of these factors become integral considerations, allowing women to navigate the journey with a deeper understanding of their bodies.

Recognizing the intricate dance between hormonal fluctuations and dietary choices, women tailor their sugar-free lifestyle to provide the necessary support for overall well-being. This stage of customization is a celebration of resilience and adaptability, acknowledging that health is a dynamic, evolving journey.

In this exploration of tailoring a sugar-free lifestyle, customization is not a rigid set of rules but an adaptable framework. As we delve into age and gender considerations, let's embrace the beauty of individuality and celebrate the diverse paths towards optimal health. Each stage of life and every gender has its unique tapestry, and a sugar-free lifestyle can be woven seamlessly into each one.

CHAPTER 5:

PRACTICAL TIPS FOR IMPLEMENTING A SUGAR-FREE DIET

Embarking on the journey of a sugar-free lifestyle is an empowering decision, but it comes with the practical challenge of implementation. In this chapter, I'll share a wealth of insights and practical tips drawn from my own experiences to help you seamlessly integrate a sugar-free diet into your everyday life.

1. Navigating the Grocery Aisles:

Mastering the art of decoding food labels is a crucial skill. During my early days of adopting a sugar-free lifestyle, I faced the challenge of identifying hidden sugars in seemingly innocent products. I'll guide you through the process, offering practical tips on reading labels, understanding ingredient lists, and making informed choices while navigating the grocery aisles.

2. Meal Planning Mastery:

Meal planning is the linchpin of success in maintaining a sugar-free diet. Drawing from my personal journey, I'll take you through the steps of effective meal planning. From understanding portion sizes to creating a diverse and nutrient-rich menu, this section provides actionable strategies to set yourself up for success.

3. Smart Snacking Strategies:

Snacking is an integral part of our daily routines, and making smart choices is crucial in a sugar-free lifestyle. I'll share a repertoire of delicious, sugar-free snacks that not only satisfy cravings but also contribute to your overall well-being. These snacks are designed to keep you energized and focused throughout the day.

4. Eating Out Without Compromising:

Social occasions often involve dining out, and navigating restaurant menus can be challenging. I'll provide you with practical strategies to enjoy dining out without compromising your commitment to a sugar-free lifestyle. From decoding menus to communicating with chefs, you'll gain insights that enhance your dining experiences.

CHAPTER 6:

HEALTHY ALTERNATIVES TO SUGAR

A sugar-free lifestyle doesn't mean sacrificing sweetness. In this chapter, I'll guide you through a delightful exploration of healthy alternatives to sugar, drawing from my own discoveries and experiments. These alternatives not only satisfy your sweet tooth but also contribute to your overall well-being.

1. Nature's Sweet Bounty:

Explore the world of natural sweeteners like honey, maple syrup, and agave nectar. I'll share my personal journey of incorporating these alternatives, providing insights into their unique flavors and their role in a sugar-free lifestyle.

2. Stevia and Monk Fruit Magic:

Dive into the realm of non-nutritive sweeteners like stevia and monk fruit. I'll unravel the mysteries behind these sweeteners, exploring their origins, taste profiles, and practical applications in your sugar-free culinary endeavors.

3. The Magic of Medjool Dates:

Discover the versatility and nutritional richness of Medjool dates as a natural sweetener. I'll share creative ways to incorporate dates into your recipes, from sweetening desserts to enhancing the flavors of savory dishes.

4. Cooking with Creativity:

Learn the art of cooking with creativity, leveraging the flavors of spices, extracts, and herbs to enhance sweetness without relying on sugar. Drawing from my own experiences, I'll showcase how cinnamon, vanilla, and citrus zest can add layers of complexity to your sugar-free culinary creations.

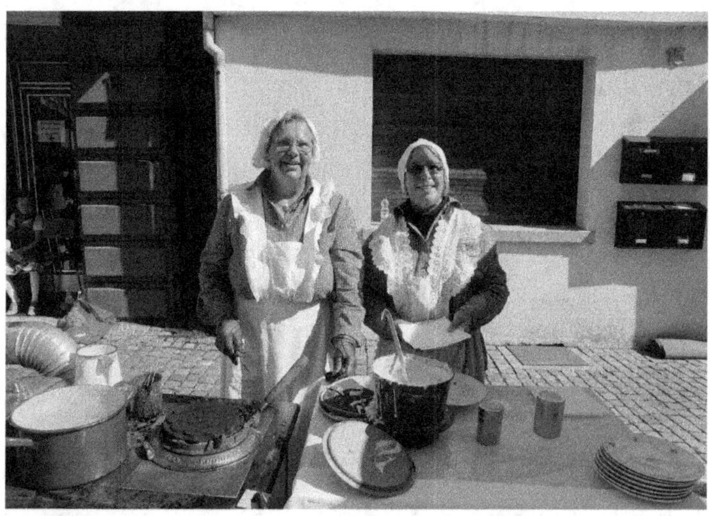

CHAPTER 7:

NAVIGATING SOCIAL SITUATIONS AND CHALLENGES

Maintaining a sugar-free lifestyle extends beyond individual choices to navigating social situations. In this chapter, I'll share practical advice on gracefully maneuvering through challenges, drawing from my own experiences. Whether it's communicating your dietary choices or handling peer pressure, these insights will empower you to navigate social landscapes with confidence.

1. Communicating Your Choices:

Effectively communicating your dietary preferences is a crucial skill. I'll guide you through the process of expressing your choices assertively while fostering understanding in various social situations. Drawing from personal anecdotes, I'll provide practical tips on striking a balance between your commitment to a sugar-free lifestyle and the social dynamics at play.

2. Handling Peer Pressure:

Social gatherings often come with peer pressure, and saying no to sugary offerings can be challenging. I'll offer insights into gracefully declining without feeling isolated. Through my own experiences, I'll share strategies to navigate these situations with confidence, ensuring that your commitment to a sugar-free lifestyle is respected.

3. Cultivating a Supportive Circle:

Building a supportive community is integral to success. I'll emphasize the importance of sharing your journey with loved ones, finding like-minded individuals, and cultivating a network that reinforces your commitment to a sugar-free lifestyle. My personal stories will illustrate how a supportive circle can be a cornerstone of resilience and encouragement.

4. Overcoming Emotional Eating:

Many of us turn to sugary comforts in times of stress or emotional turmoil.

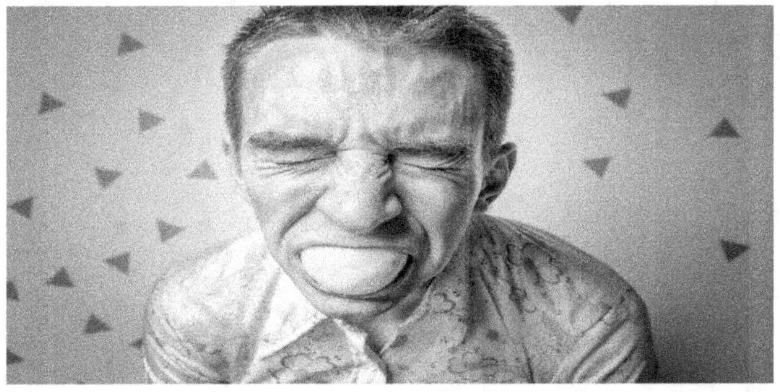

This chapter delves into the psychology of emotional eating and provides strategies to identify and address these patterns. Drawing from my own experiences, I'll share insights into breaking free from the cycle of emotional eating and fostering a healthier relationship with food.

In conclusion, these chapters serve as a comprehensive guide to not only adopting but thriving in a sugar-free lifestyle. By incorporating practical tips, exploring healthy alternatives, and mastering social navigation, you'll be equipped to embark on your sugar-free journey with confidence and resilience.

CHAPTER 8:

WHOLESOME MEAL PLANNING FOR DIVERSE LIFESTYLES

Crafting a balanced and delicious meal plan that caters to diverse dietary preferences and health considerations requires a thoughtful approach. In this chapter, I will guide you through detailed breakfast, lunch, dinner, and snack recipes, considering various factors such as vegetarianism, non-vegetarianism, age, gender, and health conditions. Let's explore the art of meal planning that embraces the rich tapestry of our diverse lifestyles.

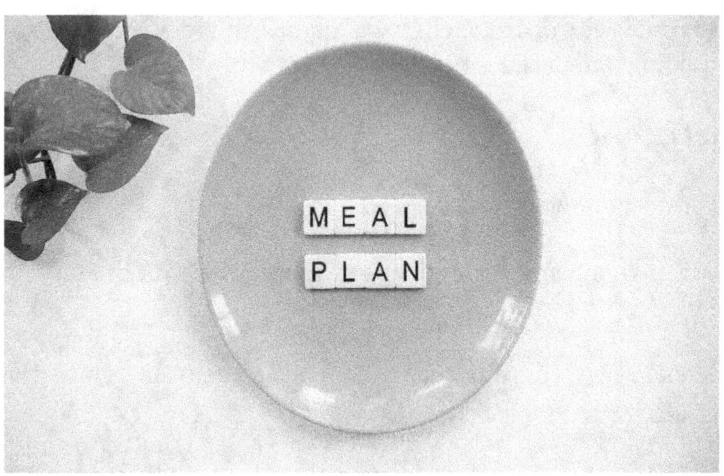

CHAPTER 8.1:

BREAKFAST BONANZA

Vegetarian Breakfast: Avocado Toast with Poached Eggs

Ingredients:

Whole-grain bread slices

Ripe avocados

Eggs

Salt and pepper to taste

Alternative toppings: cherry tomatoes, microgreens, or a sprinkling of feta cheese

Instructions:

1. Toast whole-grain bread slices.

2. Mash ripe avocados and spread them evenly on the toasted bread.

3. Poach eggs to your liking and place them on top of the avocado.

4. Season with salt and pepper and add your choice of toppings.

Non-Vegetarian Breakfast: Smoked Salmon Bagel with Cream Cheese

Ingredients:

Whole-grain bagels

Smoked salmon

Cream cheese

Red onion slices

Capers

Fresh dill

Lemon wedges

Instructions:

1. Toast whole-grain bagels.

2. Spread cream cheese on each half.

3. Layer smoked salmon on top.

4. Garnish with red onion slices, capers, and fresh dill.

5. Serve with lemon wedges on the side.

CHAPTER 8.2:

LUNCHTIME FEAST

Vegetarian Lunch: Quinoa Salad with Roasted Vegetables

Ingredients:

Quinoa

Mixed vegetables (bell peppers, zucchini, cherry tomatoes)

Olive oil

Balsamic vinegar

Fresh basil leaves

Feta cheese (optional)

Salt and pepper to taste

Instructions:

1. Cook quinoa according to package instructions.
2. Roast mixed vegetables with olive oil until tender.
3. Toss quinoa and roasted vegetables together.
4. Drizzle with balsamic vinegar, add fresh basil leaves, and sprinkle with feta cheese if desired.

Non-Vegetarian Lunch: Grilled Chicken Caesar Salad

Ingredients:

Grilled chicken breast

Romaine lettuce

Cherry tomatoes

Croutons

Parmesan cheese

Caesar dressing

Instructions:

1. Grill chicken breast until fully cooked.
2. Chop romaine lettuce and halve cherry tomatoes.
3. Slice grilled chicken and combine with lettuce and tomatoes.
4. Add croutons and Parmesan cheese.
5. Pour Caesar dressing over and mix until covered.

CHAPTER 8.3:

DINNER DELIGHTS

Vegetarian Dinner: Lentil and Vegetable Stir-Fry

Ingredients:

Lentils

Mixed vegetables (broccoli, bell peppers, carrots)

Soy sauce

Garlic and ginger (minced)

Sesame oil

Green onions

Cooked brown rice

Instructions:

1. Cook lentils and set aside.
2. Stir-fry mixed vegetables in sesame oil with minced garlic and ginger.
3. Add cooked lentils to the vegetables.
4. Drizzle with soy sauce, toss, and garnish with green onions.
5. Serve over brown rice.

Non-Vegetarian Dinner: Baked Salmon with Lemon and Dill

Ingredients:

Salmon fillets

Lemon slices

Fresh dill

Olive oil

Salt and pepper

Instructions:

1. Preheat the oven and place salmon fillets on a baking sheet.
2. Pour on olive oil and apply a pinch of salt and pepper.
3. Arrange lemon slices and sprigs of fresh dill atop each fillet.
4. Bake until the salmon is cooked through.
5. Pair with roasted veggies or a fresh green salad on the side.

CHAPTER 8.4:

SNACK ATTACK

Vegetarian Snack: Greek Yogurt Parfait

Ingredients:

Greek yogurt

Mixed berries (strawberries, blueberries, raspberries)

Granola

Honey

Instructions:

1. Spread Greek yogurt on the base of a glass or bowl.
2. Add a layer of mixed berries.
3. Sprinkle granola on top.
4. Drizzle with honey.
5. Repeat the layers and enjoy.

Non-Vegetarian Snack: Turkey and Cheese Roll-Ups

Ingredients:

Sliced turkey breast

Cheese slices (cheddar or Swiss)

Hummus or cream cheese

Bell pepper strips

Instructions:

1. Spread a thin layer of hummus or cream cheese on turkey slices.
2. Place a cheese slice on top and add bell pepper strips.
3. Roll up the turkey slices.
4. Secure with toothpicks if needed.

Enjoy these protein-packed roll-ups as a satisfying snack.

This diverse and customizable meal plan takes into account different dietary preferences, age groups, genders, and health considerations. Feel free to adapt these recipes to your liking and embrace the joy of preparing and enjoying wholesome, flavorful meals tailored to your unique lifestyle.

CHAPTER 9:

THE ROLE OF EXERCISE IN A SUGAR-FREE LIFESTYLE

Embracing a sugar-free lifestyle is not just about what you eat but also about how you move. In this chapter, we'll explore the significance of exercise in supporting your journey towards optimal health. Drawing from my own experiences, I'll share insights into the transformative power of physical activity and guide you through creating a balanced exercise routine that complements your sugar-free lifestyle.

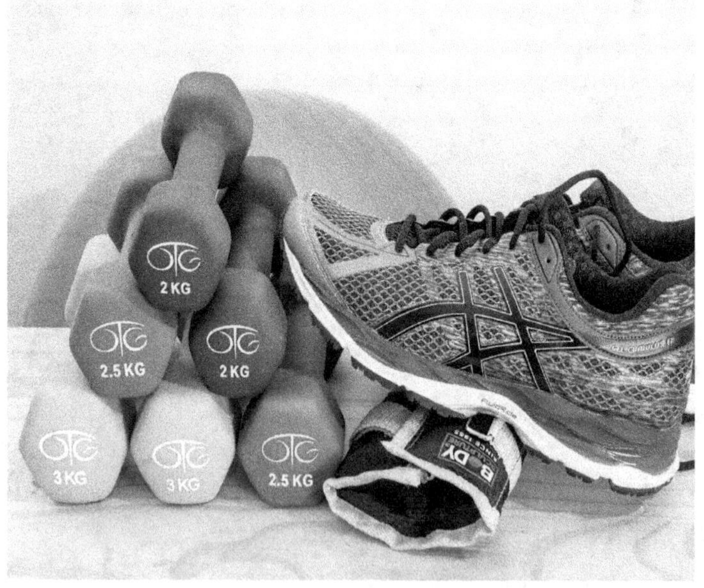

1.The Synergy of Exercise and Sugar-Free Living:

Regular exercise is a powerful companion to a sugar-free lifestyle. My personal journey revealed the symbiotic relationship between physical activity and maintaining balanced blood sugar levels. Engaging in regular exercise not only aids in weight management but also contributes to improved insulin sensitivity, a key factor in sugar metabolism.

2.Finding Your Exercise Bliss:

Exercise doesn't have to be a daunting task; it should be enjoyable. Drawing on my experiences, I'll guide you in discovering activities that align with your interests and preferences. Whether it's dancing, hiking, or weight training, finding joy in movement enhances not only the physical benefits but also the sustainability of your exercise routine.

3.Balancing Cardiovascular and Strength Training:

Achieving a harmonious blend of cardiovascular exercises and strength training is crucial. Based on my own journey, I'll provide practical tips on structuring your exercise routine. Cardiovascular exercises enhance heart health and calorie burn, while strength training contributes to muscle development and metabolic efficiency, creating a holistic approach to fitness.

4.Exercise as a Stress-Buster:

Stress can undermine the best dietary intentions. Incorporating exercise into your routine becomes a potent stress management tool. I'll share personal anecdotes on how physical activity acts as a natural stress reliever, releasing endorphins that elevate mood and counteract the effects of stress on your overall well-being.

5.Creating Consistency:

Consistency is the key to reaping the rewards of exercise. Drawing from my experiences, I'll provide practical strategies for establishing a consistent routine. Whether it's setting achievable goals, incorporating variety, or finding an accountability partner, creating a sustainable exercise habit becomes an integral part of your sugar-free journey.

In conclusion, this chapter underscores the transformative role of exercise in a sugar-free lifestyle. By integrating enjoyable and consistent physical activity, you not only enhance the benefits of a sugar-free diet but also foster a holistic approach to your overall well-being.

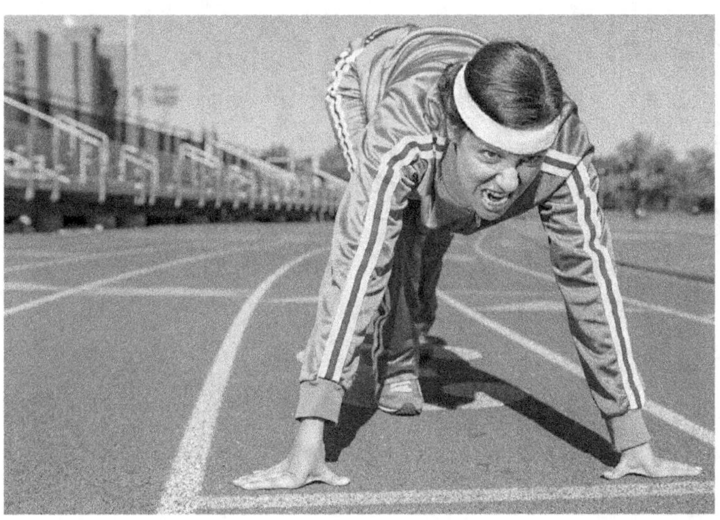

CHAPTER 10:

MINDFUL EATING PRACTICES FOR LASTING CHANGE

The journey to a sugar-free lifestyle extends beyond what's on your plate; it's about how you approach and experience food. In this chapter, we'll delve into the realm of mindful eating, drawing insights from my personal journey. I'll guide you through cultivating a mindful relationship with food, reinforcing the principles of a sugar-free lifestyle through intentional and present eating practices.

1.Understanding Mindful Eating:

Mindful eating is a practice rooted in awareness, presence, and appreciation for the eating experience. My own exploration into mindful eating revealed its profound impact on my relationship with food. By savoring each bite, acknowledging hunger and fullness cues, and being present during meals, you can transform your eating habits.

2. The Impact of Mindfulness on Sugar Consumption:

Mindfulness can be a powerful tool in managing sugar intake. Drawing on my experiences, I'll share how mindful eating creates a heightened awareness of the flavors and textures of food, making the experience more satisfying. This heightened awareness also allows you to make conscious choices about the types and amounts of food you consume, supporting your sugar-free goals.

3. Cultivating Mindful Eating Habits:

Practical tips and techniques can help cultivate mindful eating habits. From slowing down during meals to paying attention to hunger and fullness cues, I'll share strategies that have personally contributed to a more mindful and intentional approach to eating. These habits not only enhance your enjoyment of meals but also reinforce your commitment to a sugar-free lifestyle.

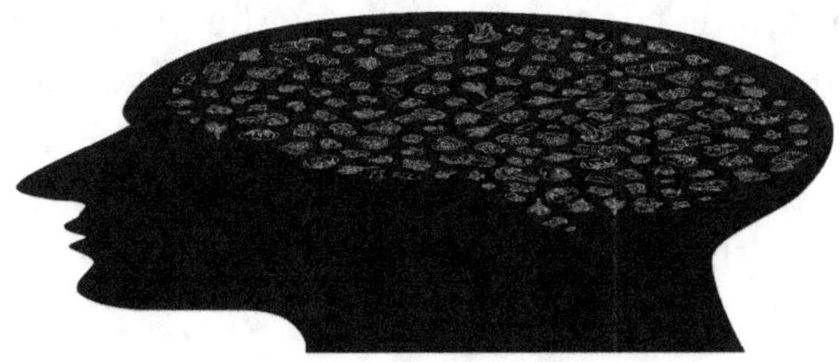

4.Building a Mindful Eating Environment:

Creating an environment that supports mindful eating is crucial. Based on my own journey, I'll provide insights into transforming your eating space into a sanctuary of awareness. From minimizing distractions to incorporating gratitude practices, shaping your eating environment becomes an essential aspect of mindful eating.

5.Embracing Food Without Guilt:

Mindful eating encourages a compassionate and guilt-free relationship with food. Sharing personal anecdotes, I'll guide you in embracing the pleasure of eating without attaching judgment. By letting go of guilt and fostering a positive mindset, you can navigate your sugar-free journey with a sense of joy and fulfillment.

In conclusion, this chapter illuminates the profound impact of mindful eating on your sugar-free lifestyle. By incorporating mindfulness into your daily meals, you can create a sustainable and fulfilling relationship with food that extends beyond dietary choices.

CHAPTER 11:

SUSTAINABLE HABITS FOR LONG-TERM SUCCESS

As you traverse the path of a sugar-free lifestyle, the key to lasting success lies in the establishment of sustainable habits. In this chapter, I'll share insights drawn from my own journey, guiding you through the process of creating habits that endure. By understanding the principles of sustainability, you can fortify your commitment to a sugar-free lifestyle for the long term.

1.The Power of Habits in a Sugar-Free Lifestyle:

Habits are the building blocks of sustainable change. Reflecting on my own experiences, I'll explore the science behind habit formation and how establishing positive routines contributes to the success of a sugar-free lifestyle. We'll delve into the psychology of habits, emphasizing their role in automating healthier choices.

2.Setting Realistic and Attainable Goals:

The foundation of sustainable habits lies in setting realistic and attainable goals. Drawing from personal insights, I'll guide you through the process of defining clear objectives that align with your sugar-free journey. Whether it's gradually reducing sugar intake or incorporating more whole foods, establishing achievable goals fosters long-term success.

3.Creating a Supportive Environment:

Your surroundings play a pivotal role in sustaining habits. Based on my own experiences, I'll share strategies for shaping an environment that supports your sugar-free lifestyle. From organizing your kitchen to surrounding yourself with a supportive community, creating an environment that aligns with your goals becomes a powerful catalyst for lasting change.

4.Overcoming Challenges and Celebrating Progress:

Challenges are inevitable, but they can be navigated with resilience and determination. Reflecting on my personal journey, I'll provide practical strategies for overcoming obstacles on the path to a sugar-free lifestyle. Additionally, celebrating progress, no matter how small, becomes a motivating force that propels you forward.

5.Adapting to Life's Changes:

Life is dynamic, and your habits should be adaptable. Drawing from my experiences, I'll share insights into navigating life's changes without compromising your commitment to a sugar-free lifestyle. Whether it's changes in routine, travel, or unforeseen events, developing flexibility in your habits ensures resilience in the face of life's unpredictabilities.

In conclusion, this chapter serves as a guide to fortifying your sugar-free journey with sustainable habits. By understanding the principles of habit formation, setting realistic goals, creating a supportive environment, overcoming challenges, and celebrating progress, you can pave the way for enduring success in your commitment to a sugar-free lifestyle.

CHAPTER 12:

CONCLUSION - EMBRACING A HEALTHIER, SUGAR-FREE LIFESTYLE

Congratulations on reaching the final chapter of our journey towards a healthier, sugar-free lifestyle. As we wrap up this exploration, let's reflect on the lessons learned, celebrate successes, and reinforce practical tips to carry forward. Drawing from my own experiences and the collective wisdom shared throughout this book, let's solidify our commitment to a lifestyle that nurtures well-being.

1.Reflecting on the Journey:

Take a moment to acknowledge the steps you've taken on this transformative path. Reflect on the challenges overcome, the discoveries made, and the progress achieved. Recognize that the journey towards a sugar-free lifestyle is not about perfection but about continuous improvement and a commitment to your well-being.

2.Celebrating Small Wins:

Incorporate a mindset of celebration into your journey. Recognize and celebrate the small victories — whether it's choosing a sugar-free snack, successfully navigating a social event, or consistently incorporating exercise into your routine. These small wins are the building blocks of lasting change.

3.The Power of Mindful Reflection:

Mindfulness extends beyond eating; it's about being present in every aspect of your life. Reflect on how a sugar-free lifestyle has influenced not just your physical health but your overall well-being. Consider changes in energy levels, mood, and the quality of your sleep. Mindful reflection helps reinforce the positive impact of your choices.

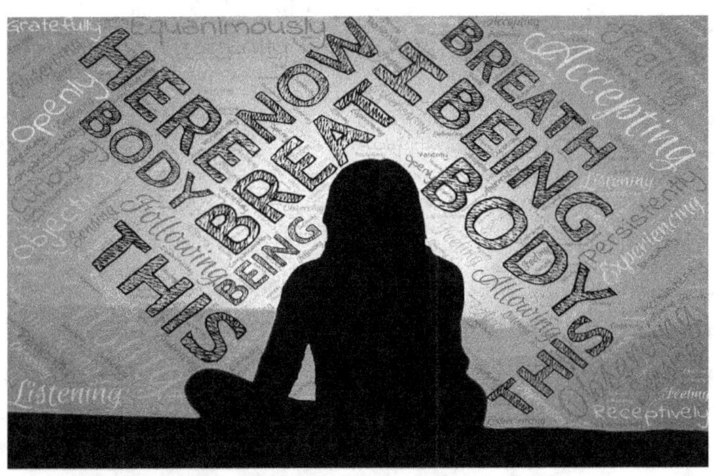

PRACTICAL TIPS fOR LONG-TERM SUCCESS:

1. Keep Your Kitchen Well-Stocked:

Ensure your kitchen is filled with wholesome, sugar-free options. Stock up on fresh fruits, vegetables, lean proteins, and whole grains. Having a variety of nutrient-dense foods readily available makes it easier to make healthier choices.

2. Plan and Prep:

Invest time in meal planning and preparation. Plan your meals for the week, create a shopping list, and prepare ingredients in advance. This reduces the likelihood of reaching for convenient, sugary options when time is tight.

3. Stay Hydrated:

At times, the sensation of thirst might be confused with hunger, resulting in unnecessary snacks. Maintain hydration by consuming a sufficient amount of water throughout the day. Flavor it with a splash of lemon or cucumber for a refreshing twist.

4. Enjoy Balanced Meals:

Create meals that balance carbohydrates, proteins, and healthy fats. This not only supports your nutritional needs but also helps maintain steady blood sugar levels, reducing cravings for sugary snacks.

5. Discover New Recipes:

Embrace the joy of cooking by exploring new sugar-free recipes. Explore diverse herbs, spices, and cooking methods to infuse variety and enthusiasm into your meals. This makes the sugar-free journey a culinary adventure.

6. Stay Active in a Way You Enjoy:

Exercise shouldn't feel like a chore. Find activities you genuinely enjoy, whether it's walking, dancing, swimming, or cycling. Consistency is key, so make exercise a part of your routine that brings joy and fulfillment.

7. Be Kind to Yourself:

Acknowledge that adopting a sugar-free lifestyle is a continuous process. If you have an occasional treat, don't view it as a setback. Instead, see it as a part of the broader journey and refocus on making healthier choices moving forward.

8. Share Your Journey:

Connect with others on similar journeys. Share your experiences, challenges, and triumphs. Building a supportive community creates accountability and a shared sense of accomplishment.

9. Looking Forward with Confidence:

As we conclude this journey, stand tall in the knowledge that you have equipped yourself with the tools and insights needed for a healthier, sugar-free lifestyle. Continue to make mindful choices, celebrate your victories, and adapt as needed. Embrace this lifestyle not as a restrictive endeavor but as a journey towards a more energized, vibrant, and fulfilled version of yourself.

RECALLING KEY INSIGHTS:

Let's revisit some of the key insights that have shaped our understanding:

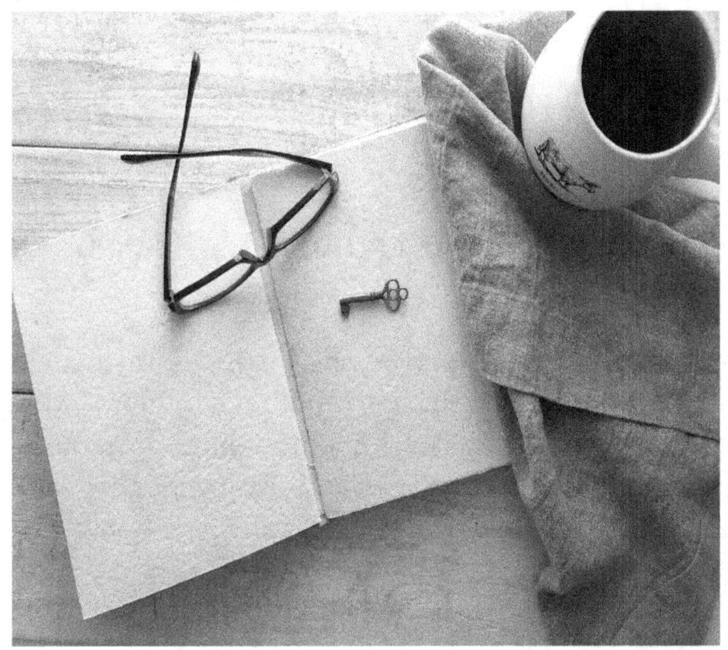

1. Sugar Awareness:

Our journey began with an exploration of the pervasive nature of sugar in our diets. From hidden sugars in processed foods to the impact on our overall health, we uncovered the need for heightened awareness. Armed with this knowledge, you gained the ability to make informed choices and navigate the food landscape with clarity.

2. Tailoring a Sugar-Free Lifestyle:

Recognizing the individuality of our readers, we delved into tailoring a sugar-free lifestyle that considers age, gender, and personal preferences. By acknowledging the diverse paths we walk, we created a roadmap that respects individuality while sharing a common commitment to vibrant living.

3. Understanding the Impact of Sugar on Health:

In Chapter 2, we explored the intricate ways sugar influences our health. Personal experiences were woven into the fabric of understanding, illustrating the transformative power of acknowledging and addressing the effects of sugar on our well-being.

4. Benefits of a Sugar-Free Diet:

Chapter 3 illuminated the myriad benefits awaiting those who embrace a sugar-free lifestyle. We ventured beyond physical health, uncovering the positive impact on mental well-being, sustained energy levels, and overall vitality. Your journey to these benefits is a testament to your commitment to holistic living.

5. Tailoring a Sugar-Free Lifestyle for Different Age Groups and Genders:

Chapters 4 and 4.2 extended our exploration to consider the unique needs of different age groups and genders. Personal narratives enriched our understanding, emphasizing the importance of adapting our approach to nutrition and well-being across the diverse stages of life.

6. Wholesome Meal Planning:

In Chapter 8, we crafted a culinary symphony, blending flavors, preferences, and health considerations into a harmonious meal plan. Practical recipes and meal ideas provided a blueprint for nourishing both body and soul, demonstrating that a sugar-free lifestyle is not about deprivation but abundance.

7. The Role of Exercise:

Chapter 9 spotlighted the transformative role of exercise in our journey to vibrant living. Personal experiences illustrated the symbiotic relationship between physical activity and a sugar-free lifestyle, reinforcing the idea that movement is not just a calorie burner but a gateway to enhanced well-being.

8. Mindful Eating Practices:

Chapter 10 urged us to slow down, savor the moment, and embrace mindful eating practices. The journey from hurried meals to intentional, present eating was illuminated, underlining how mindfulness transforms our relationship with food and anchors us in the joy of nourishment.

9. Sustainable Habits for Long-Term Success:

In Chapter 11, we laid the foundation for lasting success through the establishment of sustainable habits. Personal insights guided us in setting realistic goals, creating a supportive environment, and navigating challenges with resilience. The journey towards a sugar-free lifestyle is not a sprint but a marathon, and sustainable habits are the sturdy shoes that carry us forward.

EMBRACING THE ESSENCE:

As we conclude this journey, let the essence of vibrant living linger in your thoughts. Embrace the richness of a life fueled by wholesome choices, mindful practices, and a commitment to your well-being. This is not a conclusion but a continuation – a beckoning to carry the wisdom gained into the chapters that lie ahead.

THE CENTRAL MESSAGE:

The central message pulsating through these pages is a call to reclaim ownership of your well-being. It's an invitation to cultivate a lifestyle that honors your body, nourishes your spirit, and propels you towards a future of vitality.

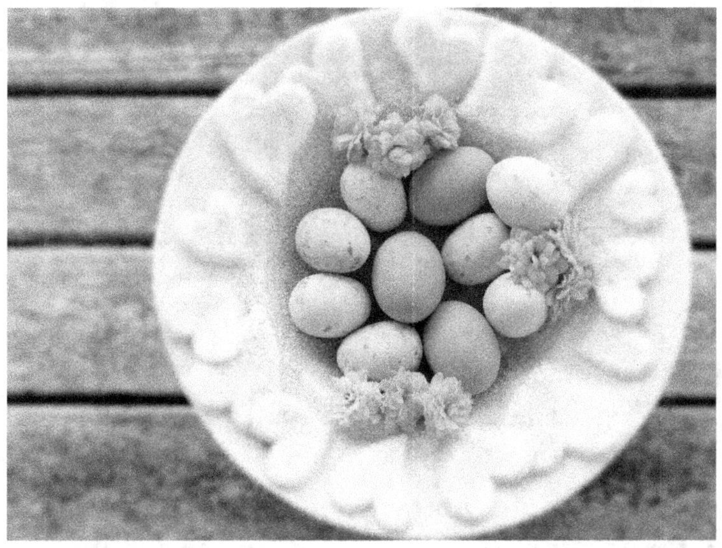

A sugar-free lifestyle is not a rigid framework; it's a canvas awaiting the strokes of your choices, your experiences, and your vibrant living.

YOUR CALL TO ACTION:

As we part ways on this journey, I extend a call to action. Let the wisdom gathered in these chapters become a compass guiding your choices. Apply the knowledge with intention, incorporating it into the fabric of your daily life.

Here are some actionable steps to catalyze the transformative power of this journey:

1. Set Intentions:

Define your intentions for embracing a sugar-free lifestyle. Whether it's enhancing energy levels, managing weight, or supporting overall health, clarifying your motivations anchors your journey in purpose.

2. Create Your Signature Recipes:

Experiment with the recipes shared in this book, infusing them with your personal touch. Craft a repertoire of signature dishes that encapsulate the joy of sugar-free living.

3. Share Your Journey:

Connect with a community of like-minded individuals. Share your experiences, challenges, and triumphs. Building a supportive network magnifies the impact of your journey and creates a collective ripple of inspiration.

4. Practice Mindfulness Daily:

Incorporate mindful practices into your daily routine. Whether it's a few moments of deep breathing, savoring each bite during meals, or finding moments of stillness, mindfulness enhances the richness of your lived experience.

5. Embrace Consistency:

Consistency is the cornerstone of lasting change. Adopt a mindset that cherishes progress over perfection. Celebrate the small victories, and let them propel you towards enduring success.

AN INVITATION TO FLOURISH:

In closing, I extend an invitation for you to flourish. May this book be more than words on pages; may it be a companion on your journey towards a life imbued with vitality, joy, and the sweet essence of vibrant living. You have the power to shape your narrative, to craft a story of well-being that resonates with every beat of your heart.

Thank you for joining me on this adventure. May the chapters ahead be filled with the vibrant hues of a life well-lived. Here's to your flourishing health and the radiant stories that await you. Until we meet again on the pages of well-being, flourish and thrive.